Clarence Doesn't Stutter Anymore: A workbook for children, parents and teachers

By Michael R. Basso and Dorothy Scarfone

I0410014

1

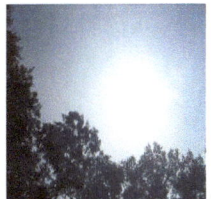About the Authors

Michael has authored and coauthored several books devoted to teaching children about disabilities.

Michael R. Basso has significant experience as a leader in quality and reliability engineering and management in industry, as well as being a college level educator in psychology at Yale University and the University of Connecticut. His experience also includes being a consultant, researcher, and newspaper columnist. Michael is the president of the Connecticut Holistic Health Association.

Dr. Basso has a Ph.D. in professional psychology and biomedical systems, an MS in engineering science, and an MBA with a focus in executive leadership and an interdisciplinary Professional Development Diploma in pathophysiology, neural systems, and education. He also holds a BS in electrical engineering. Michael is certified in quality and reliability engineering and quality auditing, as well as variety of health related areas.

Dorothy lives in New York with Frankie who has Down Syndrome. She has a daughter, Sandra, another son, Mark, and four grandchildren. Dorothy earned an Associates Degree at the Latin-American Institute in Manhattan and her paralegal certificate at Manhattanville College. She now works as a legal secretary/paralegal for a law firm in Greenwich, CT.

Dorothy was a literacy volunteer for many years starting when her children were in elementary school. She has continued to volunteer to teach English to the new wave of immigrants in her native village, Port Chester, NY. She also has been a member of the parish counsel of her church helping to establish goals for the parish. Presently, she is on a committee at her church which reaches out to the elderly. She was also a member of the Board of Directors of Don Bosco Community Center in Port Chester, NY.

Dorothy is also on the Board of Directors of the Tamarack Tower Foundation in Port Chester, NY as well as corresponding secretary for the TTF. She is also on the Board of Directors of the South East Consortium for Special Services, Inc., located in Mamaroneck, NY.

"Hhhhhhhhhi, Sandy."

"Hi, Clarence. I've come by to see how you are doing with your project."

"OOOOOOOk. IIIIII did what you said, Saaaady. Iiiiii went SwSwimming afffffttter school."

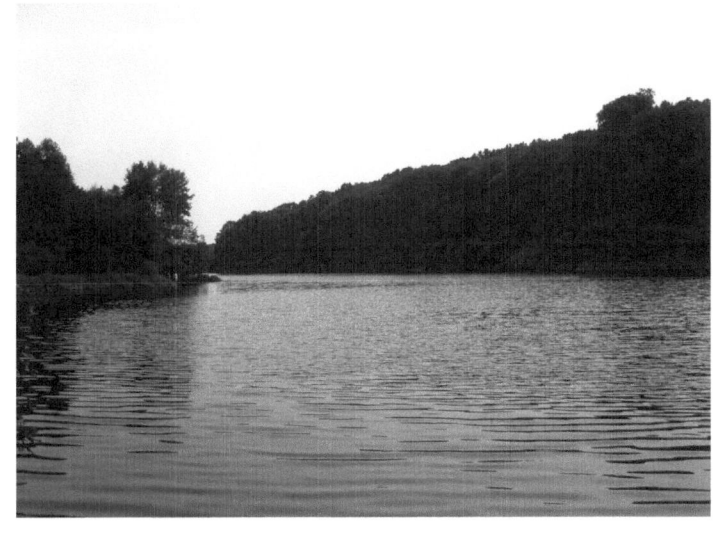

"Good, Clarence. May I speak to your mom?"

5

"OOOOK, Miss Sandy"

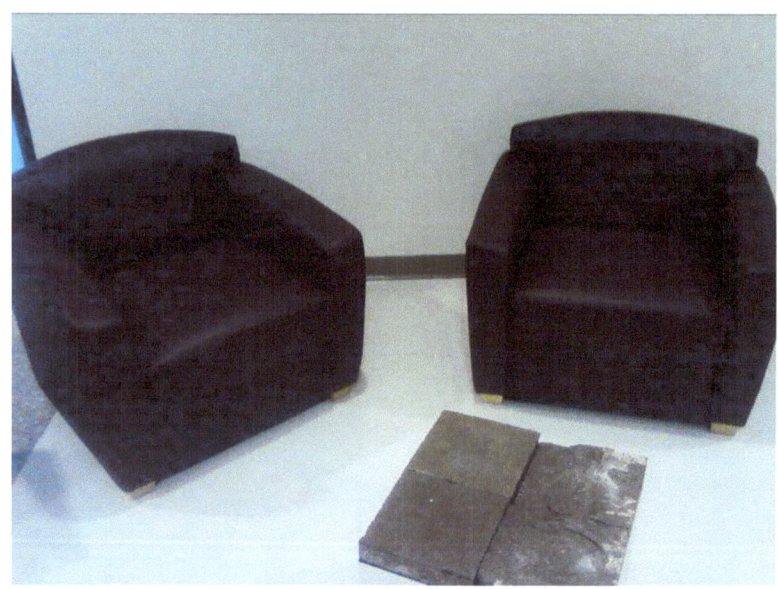

"That's   Better Clarence"

"Thanks, Sandy."

"Wow, just talking about swimming makes you speak better and seeing me helps too."

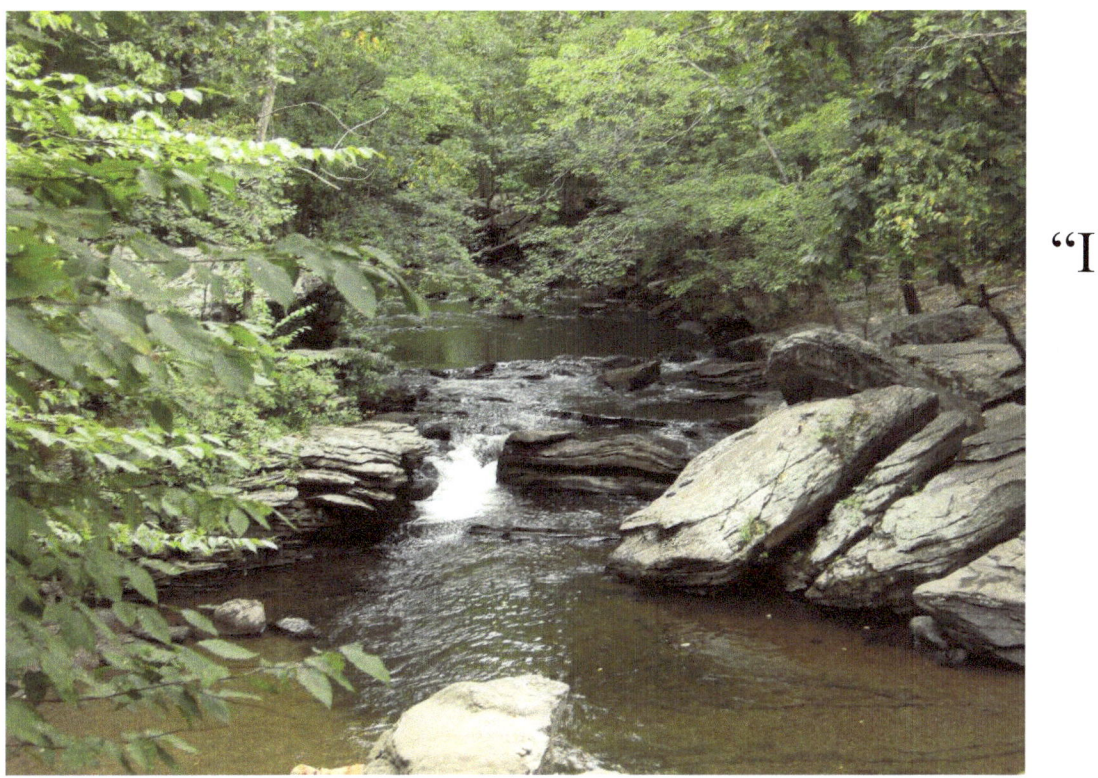

"I

guess"

"I know it does, Clarence."

"Mrs. Zelquit, your son is doing much better with his speech. The swimming is giving him more confidence. Now we need to find ways to help him to relax."

~

Mom, whee e n I play basketbasketball I can speak better too, especially when I make baskets

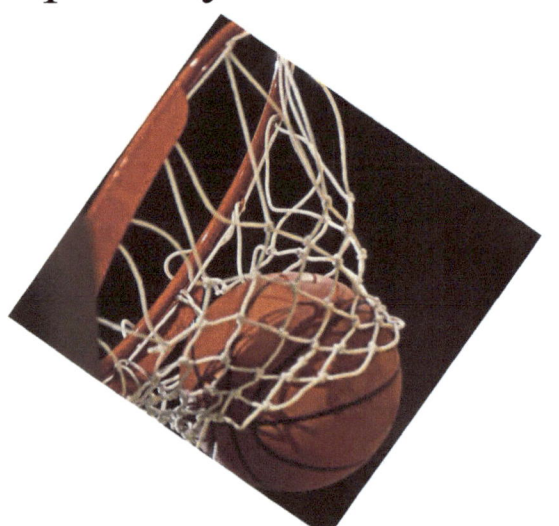

we we we wi in n.

8

"Marge, Mr. Warner said that kids may relax better if they have really nutritious foods and eliminate the sugar and the not so nutritious stuff – candy, soda, and even too much fruit when the fruit has a high sugar content."

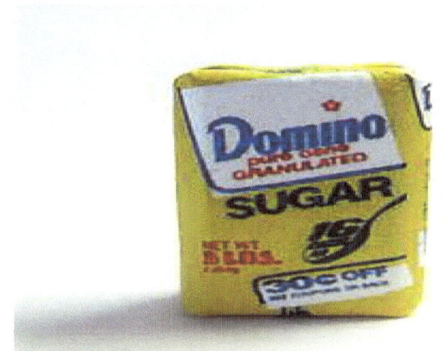

"Bart, I agree and so does the school nurse, Mrs. Pratt. She gave the moms pamphlets about all kinds of nutritional stuff like

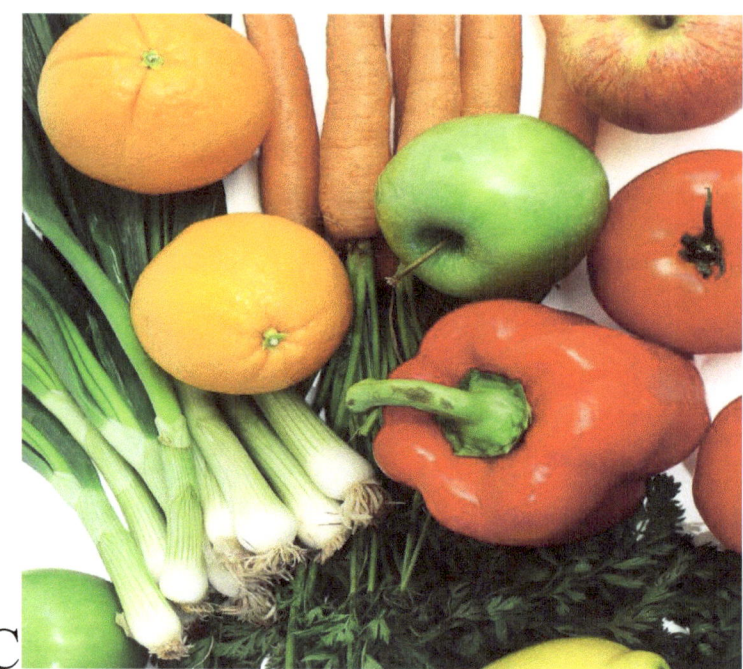

Vitamin C

B Complex Vitamins – says that balance is important and that all of these vitamins are necessary.

Omega 3 – that stuff found in flax and even some kinds of nuts.

Protein – the right kinds and the right amount.

She also told us that too much sugar, even from some types of fruit, can actually make a kid get low blood sugar!"

"How weird, Marge! Too much sugar can give a person low blood sugar."

"Bart, she said that chemicals in our bodies are used by the body to get rid of too much sugar, including urinating it out – she call one chemical

In – sul – in"

"OK it's kinda like those people who take insulin for diabetes."

"Yes, Honey. And Clarence, our son, needs all the help he can get – he's sooooo nervous and that is what makes his stammering so bad."

"Stammering – I haven't heard that word for a while. I know it's another word for Stuttering."

"Daaaad, wooooow you listened and momomorrr. You got me a puppy and a kitten and a and a aaaa kitty! You are the best dad~"

"And a fish too,

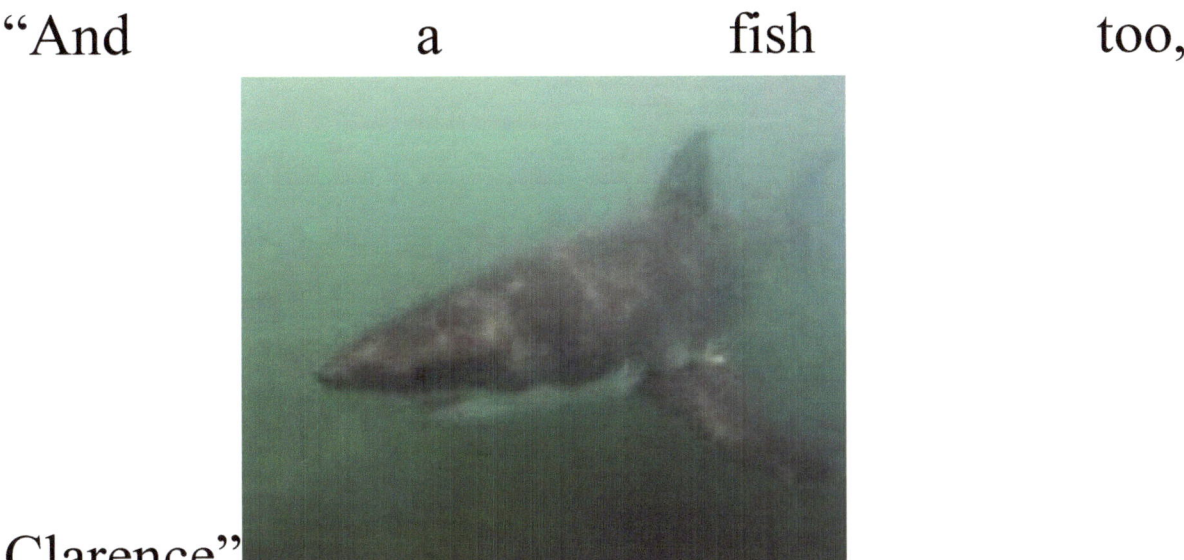

Clarence"

What!

"Your dad read somewhere that watching a fish swim or hearing a cat purr can make a kid relaxed – like meditating."

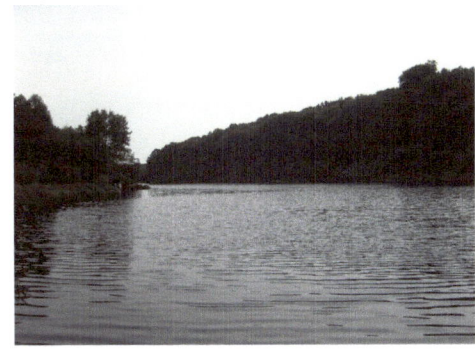

13

"We tried meditate meditate."

"Take your time, Clarence."

"Ok mom, I love petting this puppy too."

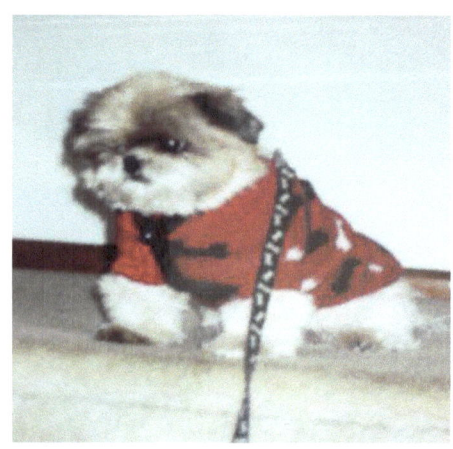

"That's perfect, kiddo!"

"huh"

"I mean you didn't stutter at all!"

"Well, ma ma mom, theeeey say meda meda meda tation takes stress away from some kids. They told us to try saying words like Om, or Hu or One over and over – but that it was not so good for some kids and and and we should talk to out par par parent parents before we try to meditate."

"Marge, says that some kids who stutter feel better when they go to church or the synagogue or temple – it gives them hope –

15

and some kids feel great what they walk with their parents."

"In the moms group, Bart, we tried to tense the muscles in our scalp and then relax them, then our   face,

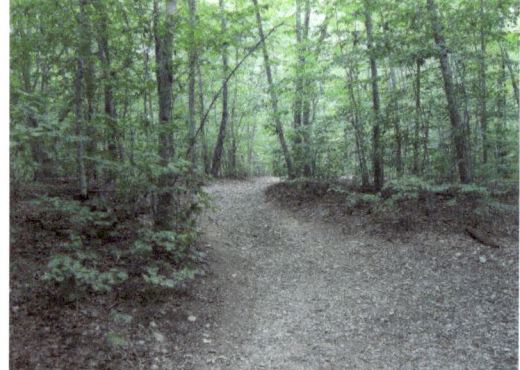

shoulders…and relax them and all the muscles all over including our hands and feet and even make a fist and even pull our toes towards our shins."

"Mom they said to never let any one touch us unless our parents say it's ok and even then to be careful."

16

"Nobody has to touch you, Honey. You can even say things to yourself – even listening to Mozart and Beethoven, helps some kids to relax."

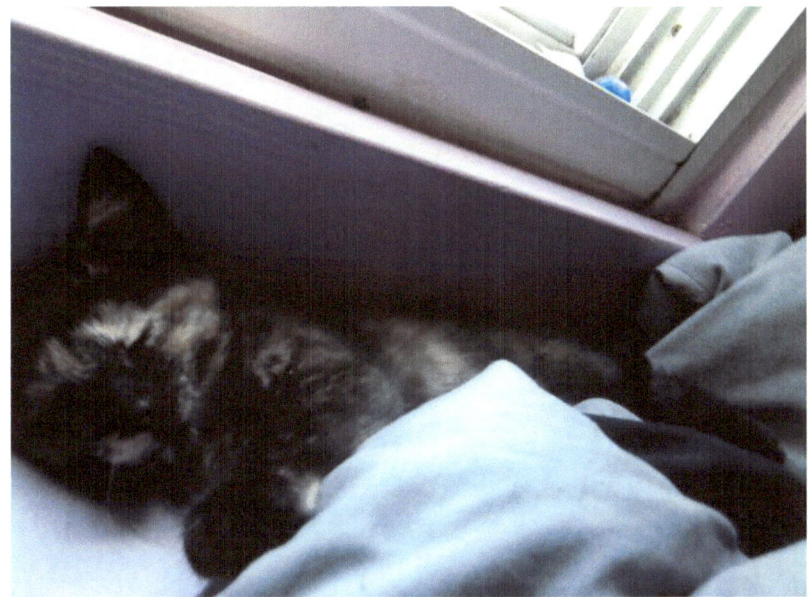

"I feel good even thinking about playing the piano and feel so good after that concert we did in school. I didn't stutter for a week after that."

"Wow! Not one word out of place – you must love hearing that kitty purrrrr."

"I do feel relaxed, mom. And my speech ther ther therapist says kids who stutter need to relax too."

"Honey, playing an instrument is like when you play ball – it gives you more confidence."

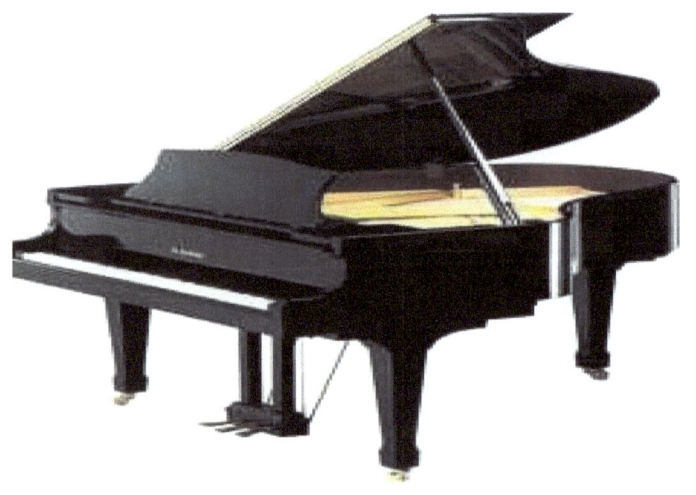

"Mom, we learned about genes in science class. My speech therapist says that some kids who stutter, stutter ah… have some some something wrong with three genes. And some kids have different shapes in their, in their, throat and mouth."

18

"Yes, those are both true, son."

"You are going to be late for your music therapy session – I told you that you could try that too – we tried everything."

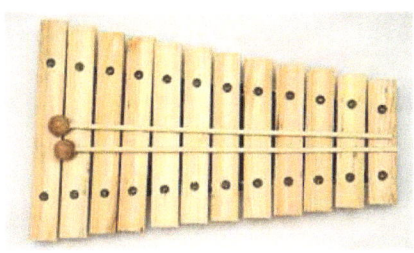

"Thanks, Mom."

"Mrs. Smith, Clarence was so anxious today and he stuttered so much it was hard to work with your son – but he will be OK. He seems a bit depressed too. That makes kids worse."

19

"Oh, he's depressed because he stutters and stutters because he is depressed. Sometimes he hesitates and blocks parts of words."

"When the speech therapist helps him speak more slowly or emphasize certain parts of words, he often feels less depressed – he feels successful and confident."

"That is a great observation. Parents and teachers can help kids feel more confident and successful and that makes stutters do much better. Criticizing can have the opposite effect.

"I know, Mrs. Smith. I have some students who get ashamed and things get worse. The negative emotions even fear, or frustration or guilt. We must be very positive around Clarence."

"When Clarence stayed few days 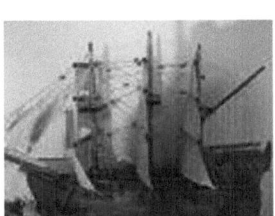 Bart's dad was ill, was so bad, he even home from school for a and then he felt guilty about that and it was even worse. We took him for a vacation and like magic he was real good for weeks and still ok for a month or so."

Workbook Section

It is Ok for your parents to help with this part.

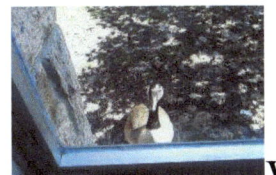What are some things that make kids stutter?

1)

2)

3)

4)

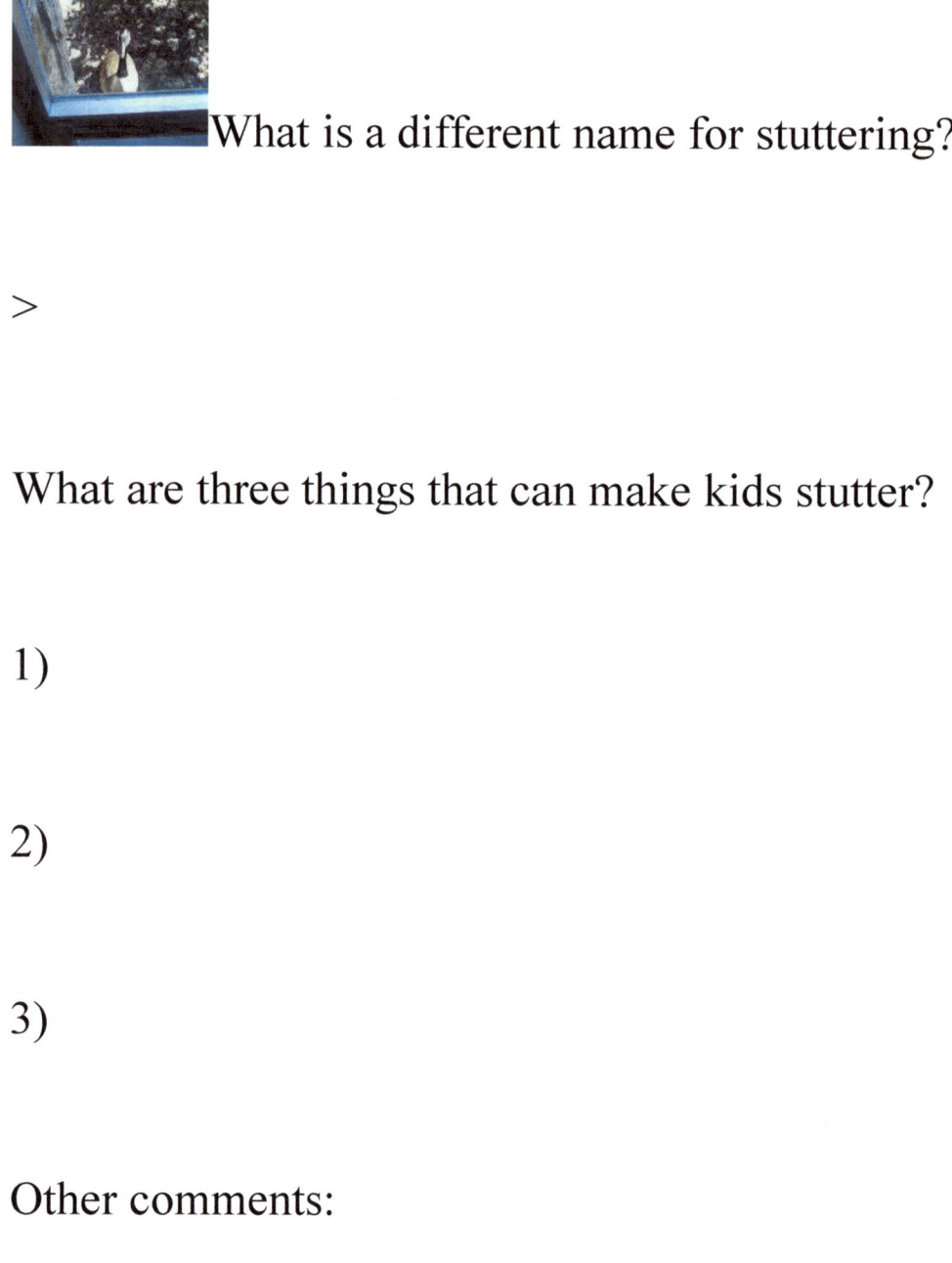What is a different name for stuttering?

>

What are three things that can make kids stutter?

1)

2)

3)

Other comments:

What are some kids born with that makes them stutter?

1)

2)

3)

4)

5)

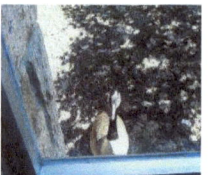How do some kids relax?

1)

2)

3)

4)

5)

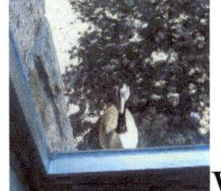

What do you do that makes you feel confident?

1)

2)

3)

4)

5)

6)

Are there things we can do to make others feel more confident?

1)

2)

3)

4)

Make up your own questions

Notes:

Notes:

www.ingramcontent.com/pod-product-compliance
Lightning Source LLC
Chambersburg PA
CBHW060805290526
45792CB00005BA/1530